Distribution, publication, and copying in any form are prohibited and subject to damages.

TEN HYPNOSES

Copying, publishing, and sharing with third parties are only permitted with the written consent of the author. Please observe the notes on copyright and usage.

Distribution, publication, and copying in any form are prohibited and subject to damages.

Copying, publishing, and sharing with third parties are only permitted with the written consent of the author. Please observe the notes on copyright and usage.

Ingo Michael Simon

TEN HYPNOSES

30
NEURODERMATITIS, ATOPIC DERMATITIS

Copying, publishing, and sharing with third parties are only permitted with the written consent of the author. Please observe the notes on copyright and usage.

Distribution, publication, and copying in any form are prohibited and subject to damages.

© 2024 Ingo Michael Simon
All rights reserved.
Independently published
www.ingosimon.com

Important Notes for Urgent Attention:

The contents of this book are based on the practical experiences of the author with hypnosis applications and psychotherapy in a trance state. Although the author has strived for the utmost care, errors or misunderstandings in the presentation cannot be completely excluded. Therapeutic work with people and the application of hypnosis are solely the responsibility of the hypnotist. It cannot be ruled out that parts of this book may be misunderstood or that the application of a presented procedure may cause an undesirable reaction in the client. The author also assumes no co-responsibility if work with a client is carried out with reference to the statements in this book.

The Author:

Ingo Michael Simon studied psychology and education and is a hypnotherapist with practices in southwestern Germany and Switzerland. With the help of hypnosis-supported psychotherapy, he primarily treats people with persistent psychological conditions. His practice focuses on anxiety disorders, pathological compulsions, and psychosomatic illnesses. His therapeutic offerings mainly include classical and modern hypnosis applications and the dreamland therapy he developed himself.

Copying, publishing, and sharing with third parties are only permitted with the written consent of the author. Please observe the notes on copyright and usage.

Distribution, publication, and copying in any form are prohibited and subject to damages.

INTRODUCTION	6
COPYRIGHT AND USAGE	8
HYPNOSIS 1	10
HYPNOSIS 2	15
HYPNOSIS 3	20
HYPNOSIS 4	25
HYPNOSIS 5	29
HYPNOSIS 6	33
HYPNOSIS 7	37
HYPNOSIS 8	42
HYPNOSIS 9	47
HYPNOSIS 10	52
ALL TITLES IN THE SERIES	57

Copying, publishing, and sharing with third parties are only permitted with the written consent of the author. Please observe the notes on copyright and usage.

Introduction

The series "Ten Hypnoses" is very well known in Germany, Austria, and Switzerland as a collection of texts for therapeutic work and is used by numerous psychotherapeutic practices, doctors, therapists, coaches, and other helping professionals. I am pleased to now be able to offer these texts in other countries as well.

Most therapists have their own methods for inducing and deepening trance as well as for exiting trance. Therefore, I have focused on the main part of the hypnosis. The texts in this book can be integrated as the main part into any hypnosis process. The texts in this collection use various hypnosis techniques. I will not explain these in detail, as I assume that users have the appropriate training. It is also not necessary to understand the exact structure or functioning of the different parts. The texts can simply be read aloud, and they will have their effect.

Decide for yourself which text best suits your client or patient at any given time. You can also combine passages from different texts. It is not about using all ten hypnoses in sequence. It is a selection of possibilities.

I want to emphasize that books cannot replace therapy. Psychotherapy or other therapeutic treatments involve much more. A careful diagnosis is the necessary basis for deciding on the use of methods, including whether hypnosis or one of my texts should be used. Even in this case, preparatory discussions, follow-up discussions during the session, and of course, a therapeutic concept for the sequence of sessions and the content approaches are essential parts of therapy. This cannot and should not be achieved with a collection of texts.

In any case, I wish you much success in your work and I am pleased if my text templates can contribute in a small way.

Ingo Michael Simon

Copyright and Usage

Copying, publishing, and sharing with third parties is prohibited and only permitted with the written consent of the author. Please observe the following copyright and usage guidelines.

This work has been carefully crafted and created to the best of the author's knowledge and personal experience. It comprises text templates and application guidelines for professional hypnosis sessions. The author is a licensed psychotherapist with extensive experience in psychotherapy, coaching, and personal training using hypnotic techniques and methods. Nevertheless, the author and the publisher assume no liability for the accuracy of information, instructions, and advice, nor for any typographical errors. The author and publisher accept no responsibility or liability for the application of these texts and recommendations with clients or patients, nor for any potential consequences or unexpected reactions. It is expressly noted that the application of therapeutic and advisory techniques and formulations lies solely and entirely within the responsibility of the practitioner. This also applies to adherence to the boundaries of legally regulated medical and therapeutic practices. The fact that a book containing action proposals is freely available for sale does not imply that its application with clients or patients is permitted for everyone.

Hypnosis 1

You are here today because you want to support your skin in healing... You have this goal of having soft and smooth skin again, just like it used to be... You want the itching and redness to disappear, and the hardening of your skin to resolve... You focus on the idea of healing because it's important to have a clear vision of the outcome... So, you imagine how your skin will look once it's fully healed... Even more than that... You imagine how pleasant your skin will feel once it's completely healed... It's especially easy for you now to create a vivid picture of how wonderful it will be to have healed, new skin... And you're equally successful in visualizing how your skin will appear when it's healthy again... This image is important and will help you...

You've often thought about your skin changes and wondered where they come from and why your skin hasn't already healed... Maybe you have an explanation or an idea, but perhaps there isn't a clear explanation, and it's much more important to focus on constructive and helpful thoughts... A special thought that can help you heal your skin as quickly as possible... So today, you formulate the positive thought that tells you... I love myself and my body, and that's why my skin will heal... And the more you think this thought or say it out loud, the stronger it becomes... The more stable the truth of this thought becomes... I love myself and my body, and that's why my skin will heal...

When you look at and feel your body, your attention often focuses on the neurodermatitis and the goal of healing... And it's good that you're focused on the goal of healing... At the same time, your body is more than just skin... Many parts of your body are very healthy and function excellently for you... And right now, you're aware of the parts or organs of your body that have never been affected by illness...

And you realize that your body has the potential to be healthy... And many illnesses, small or large, that you've had have healed... So, your skin condition can heal too... Your body now activates its self-healing power... Your body can do this and is helping you... Your body is truly beginning the healing process for your skin... Your body is really starting to heal your skin...

Body and soul are directly connected; this is always the case... The way your body feels is how you feel deep inside... And your emotions and feelings affect your body... Right now, the calmness and relaxation of your body are affecting your mood... Because you feel calm and have become tired... Your emotions are aligning with your body's state of trance... And this emotional calm, this inner balance, is again affecting your body... And calm and balance also soothe the processes in your skin... Your skin is calming down... And calm skin can heal... Calmed skin can truly heal...

Your inner calm goes deeper and spreads, and healing of the skin follows... Deeper calm and healing of the skin follow... The more intensely you can feel inner calm and relaxation now, the stronger the power of your body becomes, using this power to truly heal your skin... Now the healing of your skin begins... Now the healing of your skin begins...

Since inner calm can help you, you make your new thought your priority every day... Your thought that says... I love myself and my body, and that's why my skin will heal... And to feel every day that you truly can love yourself, you start your day with a self-hug... As soon as you get up in the morning, you give yourself a self-hug and say... I love myself and my body, and that's why my skin will heal... This sets your body on self-healing... This truly sets your body on self-healing... If you manage to start every day with a self-hug, then self-healing will also succeed... Then the self-healing of your skin will happen quickly... So, you decide to start every day with a self-hug... And you won't let anything deter you... Nothing and no one can stop you from starting your day with a self-hug... Because with a self-hug in the morning, you also activate your thought... I love myself and my body, and that's why my skin will heal...

Today you've come closer to your goal, you've activated and started the self-healing of your body... And by doing so, you've activated and started the healing of your skin... First, you created an important image of healthy skin, you imagined and are still imagining how pleasant your skin will feel once it's completely healthy again... You have your helpful thought... You think it repeatedly and tell yourself... I love myself and my body, and that's why my skin will heal... Because this thought helps you in healing your skin...

Your body has shown many times in the past that it can heal illnesses, and therefore your body can also heal your skin and is doing so for you... Your body uses its healing power to heal your skin... The healing begins now... The healing of your skin begins now...

Hypnosis 2

You have decided to do something effective against the neurodermatitis... To do something that will allow your skin to heal as quickly as possible and feel good... You have firmly taken on this goal and set your mind on healing your skin... And that's why you succeed in allowing your skin to heal... Today, you have committed yourself more intensely and confidently to enabling the healing of your skin and doing everything you can to make it happen... More than ever before, today you have set your mind and all your strength on healing your skin... And that's why it works... Today, you take an important step toward healing your skin... Today, you take a bigger step than before, helping your skin in its healing process... Today, you even take the biggest step in a long time because you are here, and you have chosen trance... This beautiful state of calm, which allows much more than you ever thought possible... You are doing wonderfully... You are truly focusing perfectly and completely on the goal of healing... That's right, that's exactly how it should be, and it's the very best... You are truly achieving your goal...

First, you realize how strong you really are... Simply focus now on your feelings and your bodily sensations, because that's how you can feel your strength most intensely... Your strength has often helped you get through tough times and remain capable in difficult situations... And it works today as well... You are truly strong, and you can feel your inner strength now more clearly... You can feel it very distinctly when you focus on your feelings... You are indeed very strong, and this immense strength becomes even more stable... Because strength helps you in healing your skin... Today, you are stronger than ever before, much stronger than ever before... Inner strength is what you need to protect your weakened skin... To support your affected and weakened skin in its healing process, and today you manage to fully align with your strong side and process and endure what's deep inside so that it doesn't need to break out through your skin anymore...

Deep inside, you find calm, and this calm is necessary because inner calm also allows your skin to calm down... The feelings and blockages inside manifest in our bodies externally; this is how neurodermatitis developed for you... But that wasn't your fault... It had to happen because you didn't have enough strength for yourself, but today you have regained strength that you can use... So now you find calm, and your skin also finds calm and heals... You find more calm than you expected; you may also feel old burdens inside slowly dissolving and fading away... You have carried many burdens with you, but they belong to the past, so now you find real calm... And your skin heals... Your skin truly heals because all burdens inside dissolve and leave you... It's truly remarkable how quickly you can shift internally, how well you can adopt a new inner attitude... And it's absolutely noteworthy how well you manage to experience this deep calm and help your skin heal... Inside, everything is absolutely calm and fine... And your skin is becoming fine too...

Deep within you lies this special strength that helps you... Your strength to resolve difficulties... To let go of burdens... To overcome obstacles... And this strength, this power center within you, now actively processes all disturbing thoughts and all burdensome memories... It's like an inner fire that gives you energy and warmth... In your power center, this fire burns, and all burdens and all difficult memories are burned there, turning into energy... This is how something good comes from all difficulties... Energy and warmth... Energy that helps you allow your skin to heal... Your skin follows your inner feelings and needs... You have this need for relief, and therefore your skin is relieved... You have this strong need to be internally free and balanced, and this need is now fulfilled... And with that, your skin heals... With that, your skin truly heals and can feel good again... More than ever before, your need aligns with your own energy and therefore produces a new healing that starts inside and moves outward... Real healing inside and real healing outside, healing your skin... Now...

You can be proud of yourself because you've taken a significant step... Maybe you already realize how important the thoughts and words you heard from me were... And perhaps you're now wondering how quickly you'll notice the first big signs of healing... You will recognize the healing of your skin because you've chosen the right path... You will recognize the healing because you've truly embraced my words and made them your own... You've shown a lot of trust and have therefore set yourself up remarkably well for healing, more than you may realize...

Today, you've done the best for healing your skin, and that's why it will become reality... Every day, you can feel the healing until your skin feels good again, soon... And very soon, your skin will feel good again... Very soon, your skin will feel much better and softer... As if renewed... Very soon, your skin will feel healthy and pleasant, soft and smooth... Just like it used to be, long before the neurodermatitis... It will be like it was before, very soon... Very soon...

Hypnosis 3

Today, you want to support your skin in healing... You want your skin to be healthy... Or more precisely, you want your entire skin to be as healthy as your healthy skin... Because you also have healthy skin, with many parts of your body where the skin is healthy... And it's important that your entire body has such healthy skin... You make it clear to yourself that you also have healthy skin; it's important to keep that in your consciousness as well... I'll show you in a moment why this is helpful... You are now preparing to particularly feel your healthy skin today... It's truly amazing how quickly you can turn your thoughts away from the diseased skin and now say: I also have healthy skin...

Now feel your body and find a part of your body where the skin feels healthy... Not your entire body is affected by neurodermatitis; there are healthy areas of your skin... Areas of your skin that feel good... Soft skin that is flexible and smooth, just as you imagine and wish for healthy skin all over your body... You find the very best spot... You now find the area of your skin that feels really good... So good that you think, this is how the skin of my entire body should be... This is how the skin of my entire body must be... Maybe there is more than one healthy and truly good spot... You simply choose the area of your healthy skin that can be a model for your entire skin... Focus your attention entirely on this spot... Concentrate completely on your healthy skin... Now... Well done... Direct your perception and attention entirely to that spot now... If you can reach the healthy spot with your hand, you can also place a hand on it to feel it even better... Or you simply direct your attention more and more to that spot... As if there were nothing else but this healthy and smooth skin... And indeed, right now there is nothing more important than this healthy skin... Nothing more important than your healthy skin... Your healthy skin... Because you have healthy skin right there... You have healthy skin that helps your entire body have healthy skin everywhere... Makes your entire skin healthy and keeps it healthy... Smooth and soft... Gentle and flexible... Healthy skin all over your body... That's the goal... And every healthy skin cell helps you with that... Now perceive the feeling of healthy skin... Feel how it feels... Feel your healthy skin... Let this feeling of healthy skin become very clear... Very, very clearly healthy skin... And now imagine that this healthy skin radiates warmth... Imagine a beautiful light there, like sunlight spreading in all directions... Imagine and feel how light radiates from the healthy skin and shines over all your skin... Imagine and feel that warmth radiates from the healthy skin on your body to the entire skin of your body... Imagine and feel how the area of healthy skin expands and takes up more and more space... More and more healthy space... Imagine and feel how the healthy skin takes up more and more area, replacing the crusted diseased skin... Imagine and feel how healthy skin spreads more and more from this healthy spot on your body... Because where your skin is healthy, strong and helpful feelings are also stored... There is your self-healing power, which is now spreading throughout your body... All feelings are stored in the body... Burdens were stored in the past and made your skin sick... Burdens in your thoughts and feelings... Strenuous emotions... There were so many burdens that it was inevitable, but now things are different... Now something new is happening... Now healthy skin is emerging again... Healthy skin for you... Because you can now better let go of burdensome thoughts... You have now found physical calm, and that also calms your thoughts... Now, in a state of true relaxation, you can also really let go of disturbing thoughts... In inner relaxation, thoughts move on, and you feel freer... So thoughts no longer disturb... Thoughts move on... And you can also influence feelings; you are already doing it... Because in trance, you can focus on beautiful and good feelings... You can make them clear by concentrating on them... Just as you are now concentrating on the healthy skin... And from there, the feeling of healthy skin flows into and through your entire body... The healing of your skin begins today and continues... It is the healthy part of your skin that becomes stronger and makes the entire skin of your body healthy... Because where your skin feels good, the good feelings are also stored... The feelings that help you heal, that heal your skin... All it takes is the idea of light and warmth radiating from the healthy skin and enveloping your entire body... Maybe you can already feel this renewal of your skin, already feel that a real change is happening... Or you just let it happen and later, in your waking everyday life, you rejoice that your skin is getting healthier day by day...

Maybe you're wondering how best to maintain this... How this can best continue, that your healthy skin heals the entire skin... And maybe it surprises you to hear that your body has already relearned and will take care of ensuring that your skin becomes healthy and then stays healthy... Your body stores all thoughts and feelings... Therefore, it also stores the path of healing... Letting healthy feelings flow from the healthy skin to the entire skin and healing all areas of the skin affected by neurodermatitis or painful, itchy, or burning changes... Your body heals your skin with your help... Your body heals your skin with your help...

Hypnosis 4

You want to stop the burning and itching of your skin... You haven't been able to influence it so far; your body simply produced the skin changes... But today you can change that because your body follows your thoughts and feelings... Stressful and burdensome thoughts and feelings led to the neurodermatitis... Pleasant and beautiful thoughts and feelings help you today in healing your skin... You have pleasant feelings now, such as the feeling of relaxation and calm within you... The pleasant trance... Now you just need constructive and beautiful thoughts that may exist without doubt, without hesitation... Good and constructive, but above all stable thoughts of healing... I'll help you today with an affirmation... With a thought that you can speak, think, and feel like a mantra today and every day...

Imagine sitting in a theater... A beautiful theater, like the grand theaters used to look... When the great dramas were still performed on stage... Just like your personal dramas on the stage of your life... With thick, soft seats covered in velvet... Very soft seats... Make yourself comfortable in a velvet-soft seat. You are all alone in this theater... It is quiet and still around you and within you... Look around a bit in the beautiful theater... The floor is velvety soft... A very soft carpeted floor... The walls are paneled with beautiful wood... And from the ceiling hangs a huge chandelier, like in a palace... With many lights and countless crystals hanging from it... And slowly it gets darker in the theater... Make yourself very comfortable in your seat, let yourself feel good in your soft seat... You look forward and see the heavy curtain covering the stage... A dark, heavy curtain hides the stage of the theater... The stage of your life... It gets darker and quieter... The light is dimmed further, and it gets darker and darker... And in doing so, you can make yourself feel even more comfortable and even quieter within yourself... Because deep calm helps you in your inner contemplation... You wait for what you can see behind the curtain... It will be something special... A thought that takes a significant place on the stage of your life...

The curtain slowly opens, the long, heavy, dark curtain slowly moves to the side... The curtain opens wider and wider to the stage of your life... And you see a dark stage... But then a sign lights up, as big and wide as the entire stage... Like a neon sign that you can clearly see and read... On the stage of your life, it is written large and wide...

I love myself, and with my self-love, I heal my skin. I rejoice in every step of healing.

Let this thought take effect, let it become the biggest thought on the stage of your life... Take it into your innermost being and let it become true there... Allow yourself now calmness and mindfulness... Calm and self-love... And now you succeed in accepting and loving yourself... Because self-love is the basis of all healing... And the more you succeed in loving yourself, the faster your skin will heal... Maybe you think self-love isn't so easy, but you succeed in loving yourself more... You succeed already now because you look at the stage of your life and see there the most important thought that truly helps you... And this thought accompanies you... You make it your own...

Deep within you, these words you've read on the stage of your life resonate, and you can look at them again and take them in once more...

I love myself, and with my self-love, I heal my skin. I rejoice in every step of healing.

... Now allow yourself a moment of calm, without having to think or do anything... Just be there and breathe in and out... With deep and wide breaths... Because with the flow of your breath, the effect of the words flows deeper into your innermost being...You've done it... And every day you can repeat the affirmation as often as you want... And every repetition helps you love yourself more and heal faster... Self-love heals your skin... Self-love heals all inner wounds... And your skin will be healthy... Your skin will be healthy... You can start your day with your most important thought and end it with it... You can start your day with self-love and end it with self-love...

Hypnosis 5

You have decided to support your skin in healing... And above all, you have decided to find this support deep within yourself and use it from there... That's why you chose trance and embraced hypnosis... You know that hypnosis is about talking to the subconscious... And maybe you've also thought about the fact that your subconscious is a part of you... So, it's neither foreign nor stubborn... Your subconscious wants this healing just as much as you do, and today it will finally begin... So, it's not just me speaking to your subconscious... Rather, my words become your words, and it's just like that, that you take these words you hear, make them your own, and direct them into your deepest being... And thus, they become your own words... They are your words that say...

... I let my skin heal now... Because I know that this itching and these rashes have nothing to do with my skin... ... I let my skin heal now... Because I know that I can truly make it happen to feel a pleasant and relaxed sensation on my skin again... ... I let my skin heal now... Because I know that by doing this, I'm taking care of myself and treating myself with appreciation... ... I let my skin heal now... Because I really want to... Because I truly want to be healthy now and forever and feel a pleasant sensation on my skin... ... I can do this... Yes, I can do this...

... I focus my thoughts entirely on healing my skin and on inner relaxation and release... Because I know that this is the quickest way to get healthy... ... I focus my thoughts entirely on healing my skin and on inner relaxation and release... Because I know that I need to become calmer and more composed... ... I focus my thoughts entirely on healing my skin and on inner relaxation and release... Because I know this is the best way to relieve pressure... ... I focus my thoughts entirely on healing my skin and on inner relaxation and release... Because I know that this is how I can let go of the neurodermatitis... ... I can do this... Yes, I can do this...

... My body is now activating its self-healing powers... And that's why the rashes and sores on my skin are healing especially quickly... ... My body is now activating its self-healing powers... And that's why I'll soon feel the improvement in my skin and the relief of the itching... ... My body is now activating its self-healing powers... And that's why I'll soon feel the softness and purity of my skin... ... My body is now activating its self-healing powers... And that's why I'm overcoming neurodermatitis for good... ... I can do this... Yes, I can do this...

... I am mindful of myself and allow my feelings... Because I've understood that feelings I accept no longer break through the skin... ... I am mindful of myself and allow my feelings... Because I've understood that it was my unseen feelings that wanted to break through my skin... ... I am mindful of myself and allow my feelings... Because I've understood that mindfulness and self-love really help me to get healthy... ... I am mindful of myself and allow my feelings... Because I've understood that by doing this, I can heal my skin myself... ... I can do this... Yes, I can do this...

... My skin will truly become healthy and feel good again... And that's why I lovingly embrace myself every day... ... My skin will truly become healthy and feel good again... And that's why I find time for myself every day, even in my waking life... ... My skin will truly become healthy and feel good again... And that's why I take care to treat my body carefully and lovingly and to eat healthily... ... My skin will truly become healthy and feel good again... And that's why I consciously and deliberately listen to myself every day to feel and accept my feelings... ... I will do this... Yes, I will do this... [Now pause for about 30 seconds of silence]...

Now lean back inwardly and let these words, which are your own, simply take effect... Trust that all the helpful words flow deeply into your subconscious and unfold there... So that the healing of your skin can truly begin today and continue every day... With each day, your skin becomes more and more healthy... Until your goal of healthy and soft skin is completely achieved...

Hypnosis 6

You want to let your skin heal... You know that inner difficulties and conflicts have caused these skin changes... You know that the itching arose because something inside you is breaking out that wants to be seen... But all this torments you and needs to be changed... And it can be changed because there's no need for this skin disease... Your subconscious can help you, your deep inner self... Because you are now ready to see what is breaking out of you... You are now ready to accept what is breaking out through your skin... So, you turn to an instance that can help you... An instance that you can believe in because it can truly help you... And my words become your thoughts... My words become your words, which you speak inwardly with me... You say...

Dear subconscious / Dear inner helper / Dear guardian angel... Please help me today to heal my skin... Really help me, because I am ready to accept everything that belongs to me and that wants to be seen by me... So please help me today to let my skin heal... And help me to stop the itching...

And not let it come back again... I thank you already for this kind support on my path to recovery and trust that you can and will help me so that the optimal healing success is possible for me... Dear subconscious / Dear inner helper / Dear guardian angel... I trust your guidance and wisdom and completely surrender to working with you and truly trust your guidance and direction...

Dear subconscious / Dear inner helper / Dear guardian angel... I ask you to find and use a new way of communication deep within me because I want to be attentive and understand what is breaking out of me... Please change my inner self so that my skin may become pure and healthy and remain pure and healthy... Please let what wants to break out of me and be seen and felt surface in a gentle and bearable way... In thoughts or dreams... In my feelings or my mood... So that I can accept and process it... Dear subconscious / Dear inner helper / Dear guardian angel... I thank you now for finding a new and pleasant way for what must break out of me and letting my skin heal... I trust your wisdom and guidance and that you will use this new way as soon as possible and only this new way...

Dear subconscious / Dear inner helper / Dear guardian angel... I ask for support in becoming truly attentive and understanding your hints and messages for me... I want to perceive and understand what comes from my inner self to the surface... With your help, I can and will manage to take good care of myself and feel and accept my deep feelings because I know that accepting my true feelings leads to liberation... Because I know that perceiving and accepting my true feelings contributes to my skin becoming healthy and staying healthy... Dear subconscious / Dear inner helper / Dear guardian angel... I thank you now for accompanying my path of finding and accepting my true feelings and really supporting me in this... I trust your guidance and support...

Dear subconscious / Dear inner helper / Dear guardian angel... Please help me to be very mindful and considerate of myself and, above all, to succeed in accepting myself... To succeed in accepting and loving myself better and better again and again... Support me in truly loving myself because self-love will be crucial in healing my skin... Because self-love can best help me to truly feel and accept my deep feelings, especially when I don't like them... Dear subconscious / Dear inner helper / Dear guardian angel... Please also help me to accept and love myself even if the healing doesn't proceed as quickly as I wish... Please help me to accept and love myself even with my illness, for this way it can pass more quickly... Dear subconscious / Dear inner helper / Dear guardian angel... I thank you already for your great help and for guiding and leading me... [Now pause for about 30 seconds of silence, then continue reading!]...

Now rest and trust that your words find their way to where you can find help... To your helper instance that becomes help within you... Because deep within, your inner self is setting itself on the path to healing your skin... On help from you for you... Help from you for you...

Hypnosis 7

You are here today to support your skin in healing... But it's more than just support... You can actively help your skin to become healthy... For this, we will take an inner journey... A journey through time that takes place in your feelings... Because everything necessary for the rapid healing of your skin already lies within you... Today it's about finding the helping power within you... To activate and use your healing and self-healing power... You will succeed in that today... I'll show you the inner path to healing... And you can walk it... You are already on your way... Maybe you already feel that you are on a special path of healing... Or you didn't notice and are even more pleased to find yourself truly on the path of healing now... In trance, many things are easier and faster than you think... In trance, much more is always possible than in waking, active thoughts... In trance, everything finds the right way... The way of healing...

Now your deep inner self is moving through time... Through the time of your life... Over images and memories, accompanied by feelings you once had... Maybe many events of your life quickly come to mind, and it's as if you're simply running the movie of your life backward... Or it's like a dark and uncertain journey through a stream of feelings... With snippets and fragments of images... In any case, it's a journey back to a time before the neurodermatitis... A time when your skin was still completely healthy... There was a time before the neurodermatitis... It may be long ago, but it existed, and it still exists... Within you... In your memory and experience... In your feelings... Because it wasn't always there... There was a time when you didn't even consider that your skin could ever get sick... And on your journey, you're getting closer and closer to that time... It's as if you're skipping over the time of the skin disease... It's as if you're jumping back before the itching and burning... Back to a truly healthy time... You don't need to make an effort, don't need to do anything special or have a clear memory... Just imagine that you arrive in the time before the neurodermatitis... In a time when your skin was healthy...

Now immerse yourself in this earlier, healthy time... Feel again the special feeling of life at that time... Inside, everything was harmonious... You were balanced and could process all burdens well... Processing burdens really well... At that time, it was natural for you, it happened automatically... Constructive inner processing was completely normal and natural... So look around in your memory... Feel where you are... At what time in your life everything was still good, and your skin was still healthy... Check how old you were when everything was still good... When you still had healthy skin... Feel in which environment you are, where your journey has taken you... And then go deep into these images or simply into the feeling of the healthy time... Or deeply into the thought of really having arrived in this healthy time... And go completely into the feeling of certainty that you are really there, in the healthy time... You are in your thoughts back in the healthy time... You are in your memories and images before your inner eye back in the healthy time... You are in your feelings back in the healthy time with healthy skin... And the feeling of really being able to process all burdens inside becomes awake... It becomes awake and strong again... A waking and strong feeling of true processing... Everything that could burden you inside, you can process with this old power within you, so that it becomes lighter within you... So that no burden needs to break out anymore... And if it had stayed that way back then, nothing would have broken out through your skin... Back then, your skin was healthy because there was nothing that could have made it sick... But then things changed... At some point, it became too much; you could no longer process everything... So, some things had to be left behind, but today things are different again... Today you can reactivate the old power... You've already done that, and from now on, you can use your new strength to let your skin heal... That's possible now, on this time journey...

You grasp your own power of processing because inner processing allows your skin to heal... You can actually grab it and hold it... Feel it and firmly anchor it within you... You feel these helping feelings in your body and simply take them with you... And with this self-healing power, your journey continues... You move into the future... You go from a healthy past directly into the future... Filled with your processing power that becomes self-healing power, you move through the present into the future... Now... Into a future with healthy skin... Now... Your skin is healthy in this time because you manage to endure and process everything inside well... Nothing from your inner self can harm you, absolutely nothing... Your skin is healthy... Your skin is truly healthy in this near future...

Let the image of healthy skin become very clear, very conscious... In this near future, your skin is completely healthy again... And with this image, with this certainty, your journey moves into the present... With the image of healthy skin, with the certainty of healing, and more... With healthy skin, you move into the present... And you bring this certainty with you... And in the present, in your waking everyday life, your skin becomes healthy because your own power heals you and your skin... The healing power you bring back from your journey... Your skin heals... Your skin truly heals...

Hypnosis 8

You want to let go of the disturbances of your skin... You want to free yourself from the itching, burning, and pain... And to do that, you need to free yourself from everything inside that contributed to the development of the skin disease... For that, you don't need to know what it all was... You can't change past burdens, but you can let them go when you're in trance... And now you're in trance, and your subconscious is helping you... It helps you let go of the inner burdens, simply throw them off, and even more... Your subconscious shows you that it's really doing it... And with that, the healing of your skin begins... Maybe you're already wondering how your subconscious can show you that it's actually doing this for you... Or you know, and you're looking forward to the sign, you're already expecting it...

Focus now on your desire to have healthy skin... Imagine how nice it would be if it were already so... How good it can feel to have smooth, healthy skin... Place your hands loosely beside your body... With your palms facing up... Keep your hands very relaxed, and above all... Don't help me with anything... Just let everything happen... Everything that needs to be done is handled by your subconscious for you... Time and again, you've tried actively to do something for your skin's healing, but it hasn't quite succeeded yet... Now, don't do anything anymore... Just receive my words and don't help me with anything... Your subconscious can and will act for you... Your deep inner self can and will heal your skin... Formulate this wish, your goal in thoughts, and tell your subconscious... Let my skin heal now... And your subconscious will dissolve all the old burdens that led to the skin changes... And all dissolved burdens of the inner self are stored in your body and now flow into your open hands... All the burdens of the inner self are now dissolving and flowing directly into your open hands, which may feel heavy as a result... That's completely normal because they are still burdens that you will soon let go of... All the inner burdens flow into your hands because their time is over... Both hands become heavy... All the burdens of the inner self flow into the hands... Right and left... And make the hands heavy... Well done... You're doing it exactly right... Your hands become heavier and more rigid... Heavy like concrete and completely stiff because they now hold all the burdens that were inside... Only your hands hold the burdens of the inner self... The hands become heavier... Because they hold the heavy burden of the inner self... And everything is good this way because now the healing can begin...

Your subconscious now ends the inner burden, finally lets it go, because its time has long passed... The burden of the inner self is now just a memory... Your subconscious lets it go now, and your skin is allowed to heal... And with that, your hands become lighter and lighter and start to turn... Your hands now become lighter and lighter because you're letting go of the burden of the inner self... You recognize this by the fact that your hands are turning as you empty your full hands... The more guilt your subconscious releases, the more your hands turn, becoming lighter... Your hands become lighter and turn... Your hands become lighter and turn... [Wait for the complete turn of both hands!]...

[Please try to be patient if it takes a while for the hands to turn. Ideomotor signals are reliable signs, similar to kinesiological muscle tests. Here we are working with a mix of suggestive instruction and ideomotor communication. If you repeatedly say... Your hands are turning... it has a suggestive effect, and the ideomotor reaction follows. By implying that this is associated with letting go of inner burdens, a connection is made in the subconscious. The subconscious confirms letting go at the same time. If letting go were not possible, it wouldn't make sense for the hands to turn. Even if the turning only happens due to the suggestion, it is still proof of letting go for the mind since it was "agreed" upon. If the mind is convinced, the goal is almost reached. Please try it out. The effect might surprise you].

Your subconscious has indeed let go of the inner burdens and made your hands light again... You have achieved a lot with this and will feel this new freedom in your daily life... Your hands are now light and agile again because they are open to new things... Your subconscious fully returns control of your hands to you, and they may feel good... You can check this... Move your hands and fingers and check that your hands are entirely under your conscious control again...

[Always ensure that the client has regained conscious and active control of their hands and fingers and can move them. Let them actively try it out. If it doesn't work, help with further suggestions... Your hands and fingers are totally relaxed, very loose. Your hands and fingers are completely relaxed... You can move them...]

Your subconscious was able to free you from inner burdens today and provided you with proof of this through the turning of your hands... Now your skin can heal because only inner burdens could make it sick... Now the healing of your skin truly begins... Letting go of the inner burden leads to the beginning of the healing of the skin and heals it completely... Letting go of the inner burden is the path to healing... Only your subconscious can let go of the inner burden, and it has done that and shown it to you, proven it to you... Because only then did your hands turn... The turning of your hands is your subconscious's signal that it has truly let go of the inner burden and is healing your skin...

Hypnosis 9

Today you want to support your skin in quick healing... This is possible with a small time journey... A journey you make in your inner imagination and thus in your feelings... Maybe you know that there are unseen feelings that have made their way through your skin... Feelings that wanted to come out and broke through the skin from the inside... But today that ends because you can and will change it... On a journey through time, you encounter your feelings... Especially the feelings you didn't see before because you were burdened with other things... But today you free yourself... And your liberation today lets your skin heal...

Now you can embark on an inner journey... A journey through the time of your life... Back to a time when your skin was still healthy... Because that time existed, and you can remember it... There was a time before the neurodermatitis... You can still remember it well... And deep within your inner self, in your memories and feelings, you are traveling exactly to this healthy time... Perhaps a long journey, because maybe you want to go so far back, so deep into the past that skin disturbances definitely and surely played no role... Your skin was healthy... Really healthy... That's the time you find... Maybe years back or in childhood... And if necessary, you go back to a time when you were only a few days or weeks old because everything was still fine back then... This journey is not difficult... Your feeling naturally goes back to the healthy time when you want to remember what it was like when your skin was still completely healthy... So, you don't need to do anything special, don't need to have a specific memory... Just imagine going back inside to the time before the skin disease... A time when you felt good inside and out... A time when there were no internal problems that needed to break out...

You arrive there, now completely in the healthy time... In a time long before the skin problems... And from there, you continue... You are in your healthy past, before the neurodermatitis, and from there, time slowly moves forward... Because you approach the time when the skin problems arose... Perhaps this journey is accompanied by images, and you actually remember... You approach a situation that was like a starting shot for the skin breaking out, like the beginning of the outbreak because something inside you broke out, made its way through the skin... It wasn't a single event that led to the skin problems, it was perhaps the accumulation of many unresolved issues or a long period of inner overload, but there was a moment when it broke through the skin... And you're approaching that moment now...

If you remember situations or events, look at them... Just let the images be there because that's the best way to let go of the past and support your skin in healing... If you don't have visual memories, just feel deep into your feelings because it's the feeling of that time... It feels different from itchy or burning skin... Because it wasn't a skin problem... It's not a skin problem today either... It comes from inside and breaks through the skin, which then changed painfully and itchily... Back then, you couldn't take care of the inner self... That wasn't your fault, nor a failure... It just wasn't possible... Maybe you had too many duties and too much responsibility... You took care of others more than yourself... Or you learned that you should prioritize everything else over yourself... Maybe in the many demands placed on you, you couldn't even feel that you needed help yourself... That your feelings needed help so they could be seen and felt...

But you had to deal with a lot on your own, so many burdensome feelings and thoughts stayed inside... They remained unresolved... And through your body, they found a way out, through the skin... But now you're back at the time when the inner self broke through, and you feel good because today, you can handle your feelings much better, feel them better, and express them... So, today, you free yourself from the inner pressure because you're ready to accept all your feelings and let them out... Feelings are allowed... Everything that moves you is allowed and can be seen... You don't have to hide anything inside... Not anymore... You accept your feelings without judgment and let them come into your consciousness... And your skin is allowed to heal... Your feelings come into your consciousness, and your skin is allowed to heal... Well done... You succeed by allowing your past feelings on this journey and letting them in... They are allowed into your consciousness and let your skin calm down...

And now hold onto the thought that all feelings are allowed... Take this readiness to accept your feelings and let them out with you on the return journey... Imagine traveling through time to return to the present, and imagine you had already allowed yourself to have all your feelings and always express them... Skin problems would never have developed... And on this return journey, your deep inner self learns to express all feelings... And your skin receives the strong impulse to heal...

Hypnosis 10

Somewhere in your imagination, there is a very special land... A land where you can find refuge... Where only you decide what may be... A land of peace and freedom... Of safety and security... The land of your dreams... Whatever you have lost in your life... Whatever you have missed... Whatever you have sought in vain and despair... Here you will find everything you need to live liberated and happy... Here you will find everything you need to experience healing... Because here you will always find yourself... So you set off, in your thoughts and imagination, you embark on the journey... You go into the land of dreams...

You stand on a high mountain, almost at the summit, far above the clouds... Below the snow-covered peak, the mountain is bare and rocky... There are small stones everywhere, and you see rubble and sand all around... And under this crust, you see the beautiful color of the mountain... A soft blue-gray... But everything is covered with sand and rocks... With rubble that lies on the surface of the earth like debris or waste... Perhaps you've never thought about how the mountains actually consist of smooth rock so far up... And perhaps you're wondering why all this rubble and rock is lying around here... Where did all these deposits come from?... You look at the summit of the mountain... The goal of all hikers and climbers... The cold snow and the cool, pleasant ice cover it... The wind blows down from the summit and carries this coldness of the snow to you... Your skin is covered by this cool wind... So cold is the wind that a feeling of numbness envelops your skin... It makes your skin feel much more pleasant... As if your skin were very smooth and supple... Very smooth and supple... If you want even more cooling, you can rub the snow directly on your skin and feel this pleasant coolness... You look down and see the clouds... You're so high up in the mountains that you can only see clouds below you... Above you is the snow-covered summit... And below the summit is this bare mountain covered with rubble... Its beautiful color is hidden by the deposits... As if the mountain wanted to hide behind it... You sit down and make yourself more and more comfortable... You listen to the wind, which tells you a story... It whispers softly in your ear... And it begins to tell...

There was a time when the mountain was still very young... Just created by nature... Newly born, so to speak... Back then, it was beautiful... Its blue-gray color, this unique rock, shone all the way down into the valley, and everyone admired this mountain for its purity and clarity... But the mountain could not remain that way... It had to withstand the weather, the wind, and the cold... This was much harder than it once thought... Many storms took their toll on its strength... But it had to stay standing... The mountain had no choice... The wind always blew again... And over time, much of its strength, its protective surface, and its beauty was worn away... Sand and rubble emerged from it... And sometimes, deep inside, there was a rumbling... Deep within, the anger of the earth built up and wanted to come out... A volcano deep inside rumbled and wanted to reach the surface... But a mountain doesn't just allow that... It tries to hold on, not to break... But here and there, the force broke through... The pressure sought release and relief... Lava and ash were pushed to the surface... Like a crust, this cold lava sticks to the surface and reminds us of the force and anger deep inside the earth... As an external symbol of the processes deep within that would otherwise not be seen...

And still, when the pressure and strain become too great, something breaks out and then settles as a crust on the mountain... That's what the cool wind tells in the mountains...

You think about how you are like the mountain, wanting to free yourself from all the pressure and deposits... It is the power of your thoughts that helps you... In the land of dreams, it is always thoughts and feelings that help... And suddenly the sun rises... It grows stronger and stronger and shines beautifully... You feel the snow-covered summit beginning to melt... The ice and snow melt and gradually start to flow... Cool water flows down the mountain... A beautiful, clear, cool water... It flows over your skin and down the mountain... The water takes the rubble and sand with it and washes them away... This cool water dissolves the crusts of lava and ash... It washes the sand into the valley... And the beautiful smooth surface of the mountain slowly becomes visible again... The surface becomes smooth... All the deposits dissolve... All the crusts peel away... The surface becomes smooth again... And that's like a liberation for the mountain... You feel what the mountain feels... You are like the mountain and feel the liberation...

You watch as all the deposits are eroded away... No matter how long they've been there... They dissolve now and flow away... The sun shines and makes the day beautiful... The clouds disappear... They dissolve... Everything becomes clear and pure...

Then you discover a path leading down into the valley, and you walk down this path... You descend from the mountain to take an easier path... Accompanied by the coolness on your skin, which feels good and better all the time... Once you reach the valley, you look back at the mountain and see its full beauty... It shines in a beautiful blue, and everywhere it sparkles beautifully because the sunlight reflects off the surface of the mountain and the flowing water... You think about how the land of dreams is a part of you... Everything here is you, so you are this mountain that shines so beautifully... You are the mountain that is freed from crusts and rubble... Because the land of dreams lies deep within you and has always been in you... I am just telling you about it...

All Titles in the Series

Volume 1: Smoking Cessation
Volume 2: Anxiety and Restlessness
Volume 3: Burnout
Volume 4: Reducing Overweight
Volume 5: Coping with the Past
Volume 6: Suicidal Thoughts and Attempts
Volume 7: Psycho-Oncology
Volume 8: Obsessions and Tics
Volume 9: Self-Confidence and Decision-Making
Volume 10: Grief Work
Volume 11: Psychosomatics
Volume 12: Chronic Pain
Volume 13: Depressive Thoughts
Volume 14: Panic Attacks
Volume 15: Domestic Violence, Victim Support
Volume 16: Post-Traumatic Stress
Volume 17: Exam Anxiety and Stage Fright
Volume 18: Anti-Violence Training, Offender Support
Volume 19: Addiction Tendencies
Volume 20: Social Phobia and Fear of Contact
Volume 21: Nail Biting
Volume 22: Self-Awareness and Self-Love
Volume 23: Teeth Grinding and Night Clenching
Volume 24: Feelings of Guilt
Volume 25: Fear in Crowds
Volume 26: Fear of Flying, Aviophobia
Volume 27: Fear in Enclosed Spaces, Claustrophobia
Volume 28: Tinnitus, Ear Noises
Volume 29: Fear of Heights
Volume 30: Neurodermatitis

Volume 31: Finding Inner Balance
Volume 32: Overcoming Loneliness
Volume 33: Fear of Illness, Hypochondria
Volume 34: Anticipatory Anxiety, Fear of Fear
Volume 35: Jealousy in Relationships
Volume 36: Driving Anxiety
Volume 37: New Start after Separation
Volume 38: Fear of Injections
Volume 39: Heart Anxiety Neurosis
Volume 40: Overcoming Resentment and Anger
Volume 41: Resolving Blockages and Positive Thinking
Volume 42: Stress Reduction, Stress Management
Volume 43: Body Relaxation
Volume 44: Deep Relaxation
Volume 45: Fear of the Dark
Volume 46: Falling Asleep and Staying Asleep
Volume 47: Compulsive Buying
Volume 48: Restless Legs Syndrome
Volume 49: Bulimia
Volume 50: Anorexia
Volume 51: Overcoming Nightmares
Volume 52: Imagined Deformity
Volume 53: Overcoming Distrust, Finding Trust
Volume 54: Processing Failures
Volume 55: Humiliation, Emotional Hurt
Volume 56: Distressing Compassion, Vicarious Suffering
Volume 57: Self-Forgiveness
Volume 58: Self-Awareness, Self-Confidence
Volume 59: Saying No
Volume 60: Assertiveness
Volume 61: Setting Boundaries and Self-Assertion
Volume 62: Decision-Making Ability

Volume 63: Success Orientation
Volume 64: Ruminating, Circular Thinking
Volume 65: Accepting Pregnancy
Volume 66: Birth Preparation
Volume 67: Spiritual Opening
Volume 68: Joy of Life and Inner Lightness
Volume 69: Patience and Inner Peace
Volume 70: Fibromyalgia and Rheumatism
Volume 71: Irritable Bowel Syndrome, Crohn's Disease
Volume 72: Fear of Nausea, Emetophobia
Volume 73: Stuttering and Cluttering, Speech Flow Disorders
Volume 74: Concentration and Knowledge Anchoring
Volume 75: Vitality and Spontaneity
Volume 76: Searching for Meaning and Finding Goals
Volume 77: Life Crises, Life Events
Volume 78: Workaholism, Goal Obsession
Volume 79: Helper Syndrome, Helpless Helpers
Volume 80: Medication Abuse
Volume 81: Gambling Addiction
Volume 82: Internet Addiction, Smartphone Addiction
Volume 83: Hoarding Disorder, Compulsive Collecting
Volume 84: Conspiracy Thoughts, Overvalued Ideas
Volume 85: Fear of Operations and Treatments
Volume 86: Fear of Aging
Volume 87: Travel Anxiety
Volume 88: Anxiety When Urinating, Paruresis
Volume 89: Fear of Intimacy and Togetherness
Volume 90: Fear of Blushing
Volume 91: Coming Out in Homosexuality
Volume 92: Charisma Training
Volume 93: Migraines and Chronic Headaches
Volume 94: Overcoming Allergies, Bronchial Asthma

Volume 95: Normalizing Blood Pressure
Volume 96: Compulsive Perfectionism
Volume 97: Sports Hypnosis, Motivation
Volume 98: Sports Hypnosis, Performance Enhancement
Volume 99: Determination and Focus
Volume 100: Encountering the Inner Child
Volume 101: Cravings, Binge Eating
Volume 102: Stimulating Metabolism
Volume 103: Bipolar Mood Swings
Volume 104: Borderline, Identity Crises
Volume 105: Hypomania, Euphoria, Mania
Volume 106: Restlessness, Agitation
Volume 107: Nervous Breakdown
Volume 108: Adjustment Disorders
Volume 109: Self-Alienation, Depersonalization
Volume 110: Ending Self-Pity
Volume 111: Primary Gain of Illness
Volume 112: Secondary Gain of Illness
Volume 113: Bullying, Victim Support
Volume 114: Letting Go of Envy and Jealousy
Volume 115: Fear of Spiders, Arachnophobia
Volume 116: Fear of Dogs or Cats
Volume 117: Fear of Strangers, Xenophobia
Volume 118: Excessive Worries, Generalized Anxiety
Volume 119: Strengthening Sense of Responsibility
Volume 120: Unrequited Love, Heartache
Volume 121: Work-Life Balance
Volume 122: Letting Go of Unattainable Goals
Volume 123: Allowing and Accepting Help
Volume 124: Letting Go of Adult Children
Volume 125: Tourette Syndrome
Volume 126: Life Changes and New Starts

Volume 127: Accepting Life in a Wheelchair
Volume 128: Understanding and Overcoming Homesickness
Volume 129: Understanding and Overcoming Wanderlust
Volume 130: Dizziness, Meniere's Disease
Volume 131: Overcoming Aggression
Volume 132: Cutting and Self-Harm
Volume 133: Hair Pulling, Trichotillomania
Volume 134: Postpartum Depression
Volume 135: For Relatives of Dementia Patients
Volume 136: Self-Harm, Artificial Disorders
Volume 137: Activating Self-Healing Powers
Volume 138: Preventing Depression Relapse
Volume 139: Reactive Psychoses, Follow-Up
Volume 140: Obsessive Thoughts and Impulses
Volume 141: Compulsive Checking
Volume 142: Compulsive Counting, Symmetry Obsession
Volume 143: Compulsive Washing, Cleanliness Obsession
Volume 144: Compulsive Questioning
Volume 145: Dissociative Paralysis
Volume 146: Phantom Pain
Volume 147: Overcoming Complaining
Volume 148: Hay Fever, Pollen Allergy
Volume 149: Sexual Abuse, Victim Support
Volume 150: Standing Strong Against Sexism, #metoo
Volume 151: Binge Eating
Volume 152: Overcoming Thoughts of Revenge
Volume 153: Detachment from the Aggressor, Stockholm Syndrome
Volume 154: Courage to Separate
Volume 155: Chronic Fatigue, Exhaustion
Volume 156: Fear of the Future, Existential Anxiety
Volume 157: Excessive Worry About Children
Volume 158: Fear of Failure

Volume 159: Ending Distrust and Control
Volume 160: Dejection, Dysphoria
Volume 161: Boreout, Chronic Boredom
Volume 162: Bipolar Disorders, Relapse Prevention
Volume 163: Mania, Relapse Prevention
Volume 164: Nihilism, Feelings of Worthlessness
Volume 165: Thumb Sucking
Volume 166: Being Brave
Volume 167: Being Proud
Volume 168: Overcoming Shyness
Volume 169: Being Able to Delegate Responsibility
Volume 170: Being Able to Show Emotions
Volume 171: Letting Go of Guilt, Victim Support
Volume 172: Processing Guilt, Offender Support
Volume 173: Mood Swings, Cyclothymia
Volume 174: Lack of Drive, Vital Sadness
Volume 175: Hearing Voices with Reality Reference
Volume 176: Confident Communication
Volume 177: Standing Up for Oneself
Volume 178: Taking New Paths
Volume 179: Confident Job Application
Volume 180: No Longer Being Taken Advantage Of
Volume 181: End of Submissiveness
Volume 182: Depressive Numbness
Volume 183: Mood Drops, Affective Incontinence
Volume 184: Mood Instability
Volume 185: Somatoform Disorders
Volume 186: Stomach Ulcer, Psychosomatic
Volume 187: Accepting Amputation
Volume 188: Overcoming and Letting Go of Hatred
Volume 189: Ending Accusations
Volume 190: Allowing Tears, Being Able to Cry

Volume 191: Finding and Sorting Repressed Feelings
Volume 192: Somatoform Pain
Volume 193: Living Autonomously
Volume 194: Anhedonia, Joylessness
Volume 195: Persistent Sadness
Volume 196: Obesity, Food Addiction
Volume 197: Parents of Abused Children
Volume 198: Letting Go and Letting Be
Volume 199: Childhood Sexual Abuse
Volume 200: Fear of Loss

www.ingramcontent.com/pod-product-compliance
Lightning Source LLC
Chambersburg PA
CBHW030506220526
45464CB00006B/2674